HAIR, BEAUTY AND BODY CARE
PHRASE BOOK AND DICTIONARY

ENGLISH-FRENCH and FRENCH-ENGLISH

By

PATRICIA PALMER

HADLEY PAGER INFO

First Edition, 2007

ISBN 978-1-872739-19-9
(ISBN-10 1872739199)

Copyright © Patricia Palmer

All rights reserved. This publication, or any part of it, may not be reproduced, stored in a retrieval system or transmitted in any form without the prior written permission of the publisher. The cover design is the copyright of Hadley Pager Info and licensors.

Printed and bound in England by Cromwell Press Ltd.,
Trowbridge, Wiltshire

HADLEY PAGER INFO
Leatherhead, Surrey, England

FOREWORD

For many English speakers relocating to France, renovating their homes becomes an all-consuming concern. Then when the occasion arrives for some personal revitalisation the questions arising are: What to do? Where to go? How and what to say?

I have set about answering these questions by trying as many products and treatments as possible myself, and by asking pertinent questions of the experts. Friends and students have helped by regaling their experiences and providing additional vocabulary.

I believe this resulting phrase book and dictionary will be a valuable aid to those living in France as well as to holiday visitors. Breaks at luxurious spas can be as enjoyable as the more traditional French holidays.

I would like to thank Alan Lindsey for inviting me to prepare this phrasebook and dictionary and for providing additional terms. My thanks also to my local hairdressers and beauticians who have patiently and humorously explained their services, giving me many tips and suggestions along the way.

Finally I would like to dedicate this work to the memory of my dear sister Mo – my inspiration.

Patricia Palmer

CONTENTS

		PAGE
AT THE HAIRDRESSER	CHEZ COIFFEUR	9
AT THE BEAUTICIAN	À L'INSTITUT DE BEAUTÉ	12
AT THE CHIROPODIST	CHEZ LE/LA PÉDICURE	16
AT THE HEALTH SPA AT THE MASSEUSE	À LA STATION THERMALE CHEZ LE MASSEUR CHEZ LA MASSEUSE	18
AT THE FITNESS CLUB AT THE GYMNASIUM	AU CENTRE DE REMISE EN FORME AU GYMNASE	22
COLOURING YOUR HAIR	SE TEINTE LES CHEVEUX	23
APPLYING A FACE PACK/MASK	SE FAIRE UN MASQUE	26
DICTIONARY	DICTIONNAIRE	
ENGLISH-FRENCH	ANGLAIS-FRANÇAIS	27
FRENCH-ENGLISH	FRANÇAIS-ANGLAIS	44

AT THE HAIRDRESSER

CHEZ COIFFEUR

RECEPTION DESK

L'ACCUEIL

Good day Madam! Good day Sir!
I'd like to make an appointment for Tuesday next week.
Could you make it earlier / later?

Bonjour Madame! Bonjour Monsieur!
Je voudrais prendre un rendez-vous pour le mardi la semaine prochaine.
Est-ce que je peux venir un peu plus tôt / plus tard ?

LADIES

LES DAMES

I'd like a cut and blow-dry.

Je voudrais une coupe et un brushing.

I'd like a shampoo and set.

Je voudrais un shampooing et une mise en plis.

I'd like a trim.

Je voudrais me faire égaliser les pointes.

I'd like a perm.
Explain to me what you want.

Je voudrais une permanente.
Expliquez-moi ce que vous voulez.

Allow me to explain myself.

Permettez-moi de m'expliquer

Please put on the gown.

Mettez le peignoir, s'il-vous-plaît.

Please remove your glasses / earrings.
Come over to the basin.
Is that comfortable ?
Is the water too hot / cold?

Enlever votre lunettes / boucles s'il-vous-plaît.
Prenez place au lavabo.
Est-ce confortable ?
Est-ce l'eau est très chaud / froid ? / Est-ce la température est bonne ?

The water is running down my neck.

L'eau coule dans mon cou.

Come over to the dryer.	Prenez place au/sous le casque /Allez au casque s'il-vous-plaît
I'm growing my hair / fringe / layers.	Je me laisse pousser les cheveux / ma frange / les dégradés.
Short at the back, please.	Court sur la nuque s'il-vous-plaît.
Do I / you have split ends ?	Est-ce j'ai / vous avez des fourches.
Just cut the fringe.	Coupez ma frange seulement s'il-vous-plaît.
Cut just above / below my eyebrows.	Coupez juste au-dessus / au dessous de mes sourcils.
Cut a wispy fringe.	Coupez une frange très fine.
Cut a thick fringe.	Coupez une frange épaisse.
Which side do you have your parting?	De quel côté vous aimez votre raie ?
I'd like a right / left / middle parting.	Je voudrais une raie à droite / à gauche / au milieu.
I don't like my ears showing.	Je n'aime pas que mes oreilles soient dégagés.
Can you layer my hair?	Pouvez-vous dégrader mes cheveux ?
You have a high crown.	Vous avez le sommet du crâne haut.
I'd like / don't like gel / lacquer.	Je voudrais /je n'aime pas le gel /la laque.
Please use /don't use the razor.	Utilisez / n'utilisez pas le rasoir s'il-vous-plaît.
I have dyed hair.	J'ai les cheveux teints.
I dye my hair.	Je me teins les cheveux.
I'd like my roots re-coloured.	Je voudrais une recoloration de mes racines.
I'd like my hair highlighted.	Je voudrais des mèches.
How much are highlights?	Combien ça coûte les mèches ?
I'd like blond highlights.	Je voudrais des mèches blondes.
I'd like two or three colour highlights.	Je voudrais des mèches avec deux ou trois couleurs.

Do I have a lot of grey hairs?	Est-ce que j'ai beaucoup de cheveux gris ?
I'd like an all over colour.	Je voudrais une couleur uniforme mais je voudrais une couleur differente,
and with a few lighter streaks / highlights.	et avec quelques mèches / ou un lèger balayage.
The product is burning my skin / scalp.	Le produit me brûle ma peau / mon cuir chevelu / ma tête.
I'd like a loose / tight perm.	Je voudrais une mini-vague / permanente.
How long will the treatment take?	Combien de temps prendra le traitement ? / Combien de temps cela dure ?
I'm very happy, thank you.	Je suis très contente, merci.
I admit, I'm disappointed.	Je m'avoue déçue / Je suis déçue.
This shampoo has ruined my hair!	Ce shampooing a abîmé mes cheveux !
I'm seething (with anger).	Je bous de colère / Je suis en colère – ma coiffure me plaît pas.
Where's my coat / jacket, please?	Où est mon manteau / ma veste s'il-vous-plaît ?
Ask at the reception desk.	Demandez à l'accueil.
I'd like to give you a tip.	Je voudrais vous donner un pourboire.
Our staff don't accept tips / gratuities.	Pourboire interdit pour nos personelles / pour le personnel (ou) pour notre personnel.

RECEPTION DESK	**L'ACCUEIL**
Sorry, I have no change.	Je regrette, je n'ai pas de monnaie.
We accept payment by cheque or credit card.	Nous acceptons les versements par chèque ou carte de crédit.

MEN

I'd like a haircut please.

Don't cut it too short.
A little more off the back and sides please.
Short back-and-sides, please.

Please trim my moustache.

I'd like you to shave off my beard, please.
I always put on aftershave.

I'd like some hair extensions.

LES HOMMES

Je voudrais me faire couper les cheveux s'il-vous-plaît.
Pas trop court.
Dégager un peu plus derrière et sur les côtés.
Coupez très court derrière et sur les côtés, s'il-vous-plaît.

Pourriez-vous me refraîchir la moustache.

Je voudrais raser ma barbe s'il-vous-plaît.
Je me mets toujours de l'après-rasage.

Je voudrais des extensions s'il-vous-plaît.

AT THE BEAUTICIAN

Good day Madam.
Can I help you?
Can you help me, please?

Thank you for your help.

I'd like a facial.
I'd like a manicure.
I'd like a massage.
I'd like a neck and back massage.

À L'INSTITUT DE BEAUTÉ CHEZ L'ESTHÉTICIENNE

Bonjour Madame.
Puis-je vous aider?
Est-ce que vous pouvez m'aider, s'il-vous-plaît ?

Je vous remercie de votre aide.

Je voudrais des soins de visage.
Je voudrais une manucure.
Je voudrais un massage.
Je voudrais un massage du cou et du dos.

I'd like a body massage.	Je voudrais un massage du corps.
I'd like a waxing.	Je voudrais une épilation à la cire.
I'd like some information about / your products / your treatments.	Je voudrais des renseignments sur vos produits/vos traitements.
What cream do you use for your skin?	Quel produit utilisez-vous pour la peau ?
For care of the complexion we use ….	Pour les soins du visage nous utilisons les produits …..
For hair / nail care we use …..	Pour les soins de la chevelure / des ongles nous utilisons ….
Do I need an appointment?	Il faut que j'ai un rendez-vous ?

HAND CARE — SOINS DE MAINS

I'd like a manicure.	Je voudrais une manucure.
I'd like a 'French' manicure.	Je voudrais une 'French Manucure'.
Do you bite your nails?	Vous rongez-vous les ongles ?
When I'm nervous, I bite my nails.	Quand je suis nerveuse, je me ronge les ongles.
My nails break / flake easily.	Mes ongles cassent / se dédoublent facilement.
I like my nails in an oval / square-cut shape.	J'aime mes ongles taillés en ovale / en carré.
Make sure that the nails are clean and dry.	S'assurer que les ongles sont propres et secs.
I'd like a hand massage.	Je voudrais un massage des mains.

FACE CARE — SOINS DE VISAGE

I'd like a facial.	Je voudrais des soins de visage.

I'd like an essential oils face massage.	Je voudrais un soin du visage aux huiles essentielles.
Please put on the gown.	Mettez le peignoir, s'il-vous-plaît.
Is that comfortable?	Est-ce confortable?
Are you allergic to any products?	Etes-vous allergique à quelques produits?
You have dry skin.	Vous avez la peau déssechée.
I have dry / greasy / combination skin.	J'ai une peau séche / grasse / mixte.
I'm using a firm and lift fluid / an intensive anti-wrinkle serum.	J'utilisais un fluide raffermissant liftant /un sérum anti-rides intensif.
Do you use face and eye night care?	Utilisez-vouz un soin de nuit pour le visage et pour les yeux?
This treatment unblocks pores.	Ce traitement libère les pores.
Show me how to use it, please.	Montrez-moi comment m'en servir, s'il-vous-plaît.
Leave the hot oil facial mask on for 10-15 minutes then rinse off.	Laisser agir le masque à l'huile chaude 10-15 minutes, puis rincer.
It has revitalising properties.	Il a les propriétés revitalisantes.
I want to wipe my hands. Is there a towel, please?	Je veux m'essuyer les mains. Est-ce qu'il y a une serviette, s'il-vous-plaît ?

HAIR REMOVAL   LES ÉPILATIONS

I'd like a waxing	Je voudrais une épilation à la cire
Full arm / lower arm	Bras / avant bras
Armpits	Aisselles
Eyebrows / Upper lip / Chin	Sourcil / Lèvres / Menton
Bikini line / Brazilian bikini	Maillot simple / Maillot brésilien
I'd like my eyebrows reshaped.	J'aimerais me faire épiler (légèrement) les soucils.
I'd like a permanent tint on my	Je voudrais une teinte

eyelashes / eyebrows.

Is it skin disease or skin cancer?
It's only skin deep.

permanenté pour mes cils / sourcils.

Est-ce une maladie de la peau ou le cancer de la peau ?
Ça ne va pas bien loin

FOOT CARE

To have a pedicure.

I'd like a pedicure
Take off your shoes and socks.

Put on your shoes and socks.

I'd like foot reflexology.

Show me your special footcare treatments.
That is sensitive / ticklish.
You have to relax.

MASSAGE (*see also above*)

I'd like a massage.
I'd like a neck and back massage.
I'd like a body massage.

Get undressed please but leave on your undies.
Take off your ……..and sit down here, please.

SOINS DE PIED

Se faire soigner les pieds / Avoir un soin pédicure.

Je voudrais un pédicure.
Enlevez vos chaussures et vos chaussettes.

Remettez vos chaussures et vos chaussettes.

Je voudrais une réflexologie plantaire.

Montrez-moi vos soins spéciaux des pieds.
C'est sensible / sa chatouille.
Il faut que vous vous détendiez.

MASSAGE (*voir aussi au-dessus*)

Je voudrais un massage.
Je voudrais un massage du cou et du dos.
Je voudrais un massage du corps

Déshabillez-vous, s'il-vous-plaît mais laissez votre lingerie.
Enlevez votre / vos ………et installez-vous par ici, s'il-vous-plaît.

OTHER TREATMENTS

I'd like to lose weight, what treatments / products are available?
How much will it cost?

How long will it /the treatment take?

I'd like a revitalizing leg treatment.
I'd like to have a face-lift.
I'd like to try acupuncture.

Will the needles hurt ?

Can you remove this tattoo?

The product is burning my skin.
That hurts !
I hope I haven't hurt you?

I'd like to try skin peeling and plastic surgery.
You should cut down on drink and stop smoking!
I don't care if you're right or not.
I don't care what people think!

AUTRES TRAITMENTS

Je voudrais perdre du poids, quel est le choix de traitements/produits ?
Ça coûtera combien ? C'est combien ?
Il faut combien de temps ? Combien de temps prendra / durera le traitement ?
Je voudrais un soin revitalisant pour les jambes légères.
J'aimerai avoir un lifting.
Je voudrais essayer l'acuponcture.
Est-ce que les aiguilles feront mal ?
Pouvez-vous enlever ce tatouage ?
Le produit me brûle ma peau.

Ça fait mal !
J'espère que je ne vous ai pas fait mal / blessé ?
Je voudrais essayer le peeling et la chirurgie esthétique.
Vous devriez boire moins et arrêter de fumer!
Je me moque que tu aies raison.
Je me moque du qu'en-dira-t-on

AT THE CHIROPODIST

Note: Chiropody includes the treatment of minor foot complaints.
Are you in good health? Any

CHEZ LE/LA PÉDICURE

Note: La podologie compris le traitement des problèmes mineurs aux pieds.
Êtes-vous en bonne santé? Pas

problems? Illnesses?	des maladies?
I am diabetic.	Je suis diabétique.
I broke my ankle recently.	Je me suis cassée ma cheville récemment.
I'm on my feet all day.	Je suis debout toute la journée.
My foot hurts. I can't walk.	J'ai mal au pied. Je ne peux pas marcher.
To put one's feet up.	S'etendre / s'asseoir pour se reposer un peu.
Put your foot on the footstool / foot rest.	Posez votre pied sur le tabouret / le repose-pieds.
I have a verruca.	J'ai une verrue plantaire.
Yes. You also have: a corn	Oui. Aussi, vous avez un cor,
A bunion	Un oignon,
Chilbains	Les engelures,
An in-growing toenail.	Un ongle incarné.
I have athlete's foot, and a callus/ hard skin.	J'ai une mycose au pied, un cal (un durillon, une callosité).
My feet are ticklish.	Mes pieds me chatouillent.
Put your foot in the foot bath.	Placez votre pied dans le bain de pieds.
I can offer foot reflexology and special footcare treatments.	Je peux vous offrir une réflexologie plantaire et des soins spéciaux des pieds.
I'd like a foot spa and treatment for cracked skin.	Je voudrais une thalasso et un soin pour les pieds craquelés.
I'd like a foot spa and treatment for sweaty feet.	Je voudrais une thalasso et un soin pour la transpiration des pieds.
Do you have a corn plaster?	Avez-vous un pansement pour cors?
To cut one's nails.	Se couper les ongles.
To have a pedicure.	Se faire soigner les pieds / une pédicure.
See also At The Beautician's.	Voir aussi Chez L'Esthéticienne

AT THE HEALTH SPA
AT THE MASSEUSE

À LA STATION THERMALE
CHEZ LE MASSEUR
CHEZ LA MASSEUSSE

I'd like to know about your facilities, treatments and packages.

Je voudrais savoir vos équipements, cures et forfaits.

I heard about you from a friend.

Je vous connais par mon ami(e).

I want to know more about it.

Je veux en savoir davantage.

I'm interested in the indoor pool / outdoor pool.

Je m'intéresse à la piscine intérieure / la piscine extérieure.

I'm interested in the spa / the whirlpool bath.

Je m'intéresse à la station thermale / au bain bouillonnant.

I'm interested in the fitness centre.

Je m'intéresse aux équipements de fitness.

I'm interested in the massage facilities.

Je m'intéresse à la cabine de massage.

I'm interested in anti-stress / anti-ageing treatment.

Je m'intéresse à l'anti-stress / l'anti-âge traitement.

Our well-trained staff guarantee you personal service.

Nos personnels qualifiés vous garantissent un service individuel.

Please put on the gown.

Mettez le peignoir, s'il vous plaît.

I'd like a sauna / I'd like a steam bath.

Je voudrais un sauna / bains de vapeur.

You will relax in a quiet, calming atmosphere.

Vous vous ressourcerez dans une atmosphère très calme.

I feel totally relaxed!

Je me sens détendu totalement!

Everything is OK, thanks.

Tout va bien, merci!

I don't feel well.

Je ne me sens pas bien.

I feel dizzy / faint.

Je suis pris(e) de vertiges / d'un malaise.

The heat has got to me.
May I sit down ?

Je suis abattu(e) par la chaleur
Je peux m'asseoir?

Yes, sit down, please.	Oui, asseyez-vous, s'il vous plaît.
I'll bring you some water.	Je vous apporte de l'eau.
I'd like to lose weight, what treatments are available?	Je voudrais perdre du poids, quel est le choix de traitements?
How much do you weigh?	Combien est-ce que tu pèses?
My Goodness, I have gained weight!	Mon Dieu, j'ai grossi!
I'm trying to get thinner. I'm on a diet.	J'essaie de mincer. Je suis au régime.
You've lost weight! How many kilos have you lost?	Vous avez fondu! Combien de kilos avez-vous perdus?
I've lost three kilos.	J'ai maigri de trois kilos.
It's up to you.	Ça dépend de toi.

MASSAGE

I have a painful neck / shoulder. I'd like a massage.	J'ai mal au cou / à l'épaule. Je voudrais un massage.
We offer various massage treatments. For example:-	Nous offrons divers traitements de massages. Par exemple:
Spinal manipulation by a qualified professional.	Les manipulations de la colonne vertébrale par un professionnel de santé qualifié.
Shiatsu massage.	Massage Shiatsu.
Shiatsu hot stone therapy.	Massage aux pierres chaudes.
Hot and cold stone massage.	Massage aux pierres chaudes et froides.
Pregnancy massage.	Massage pour femmes enceintes.
Full body massage.	Massage du corps.
Full body, four-handed, head-to toe massage.	Massage du corps à quatre mains.
Tension relief massage.	Massage anti-stress.
Essential oils massage.	Soin du visage aux huiles essentielles.
Sport massage.	Massage sportif.

Indian head massage.	Massage indien de la tête.
Hand massage.	Massage des mains.
Anti-cellulitis massage.	Massage anti-cellulite.
In the massage room.	Dans la cabine de massage.
In the underwater massage bath / whirlpool.	Dans le bassin à remous d'eau chaude / le bain de massage/ le bain bouillonnant.
We also offer a wide range of made-to measure treatments - for example:-	Nous offrons aussi une gamme de soins du corps / sur mesure – par exemple:-
Aromatherapy uses essential oils for massages or baths.	L'Aromathérapie utilise les huiles essentielles pour les massages ou les bains.
Exfoliation is circular massaging of products to help eliminate dead skin cells, leaving soft skin. It enhances blood circulation.	L'Exfoliation est un massage circulaire de produits pour l'extraction des cellules mortes de la peau. Elle active la micro circulation.
Fangotherapy uses warm sea muds to relax muscles and joints.	La Fangothérapie est l'utilisation de boues marines pour permettre une décontraction totale des muscles et des articulations.
Reflexology is manual pressure on different zones of the feet and hands to reduce tension in corresponding parts of the body.	La Réflexlogie est exercée par pression sur des zones (pieds et mains) pour dénouer les tensions correspondant à certains organes /parties du corps.
Shiatsu is needle-less acupuncture by massaging energy points.	Le Shiatsu est le massage exerçant des pressions sur les points d'énergie.
Stonetherapy is the application of stones on the body's energy points to encourage lymphatic drainage and muscle relaxation.	Le Stonethérapie est l'application de pierres chaudes sur les points d'énergie du corps et facilite le drainage et détend les muscles.
Thalassotherapy is the use of the beneficial effects of sea	La Thalossothérapie est l'utilisation des bienfaits de

water.	l'eau de mer.
Thermalism is the use of natural mineral waters.	Le Thermalisme est l'utilisation d'eaux minérales naturelles.
Wrappings is the application of products to encourage the elimination of toxins. Some wrappings help with slimming.	Les Enveloppements sont l'application de produits pour permettre d'éliminer les toxines. Certains produits aident l'amaigrissement.
All you have to do is choose!!	Vous n'avez qu'à choisir!! / Choisissez!
Here is the sauna.	Ici le sauna. (Le bain de vapeur findlandais).
The mixed sauna.	Le sauna mixte.
The sauna stove and the sauna stones.	Le four de l'étuve humide et les galets (les pierres poreuses).
Birch twigs for beating the skin.	Les verges de bouleau pour se flageller.
The after-sauna cooling room.	La salle de refroidissement après la séance de sauna.

HAIR REMOVAL — L'ÉPILATION

Half / lower leg / thigh.	Demi jambes / la cuisse.
Full leg.	Jambes completes.
Lower arm.	Avant bras.
Full arm.	Bras.
Eyebrows / Upper lip / Chin.	Sourcil / Lèvres / Menton.
Bikini Line / Armpits.	Maillot simple / Aisselle.

TANNING — LE BRONZAGE

Try the solarium!	Essayez le solarium artificiel! (Le bronzage artificiel).
The sun bed.	Le fauteuil de relaxation.
The sunray lamp; sun lamp.	Le soleil artificiel. Les lampes – à bronzer / à rayons ultraviolets / solaires.
I'd like a spray tan.	Je voudrais un bronzage par brumisation.

AT THE FITNESS CLUB
AT THE LEISURE CENTRE
AT THE GYMNASIUM

What is avalable at the Fitness Centre?

We have a swimming pool, badminton, tennis, a gymnasium and saunas.
You can choose the activity which interests you.
There are numerous and very varied collective courses.
I would like to follow a course that will put me in good form.
I would like to take a course in aquatic physical training.
What exercise machines do you have in the gymnasium?
We have a wide range of machines.
You can reserve the exercise machines at the reception.

Barbell
Chest Expander
Dumbbell
Exercise Cycle
Handgrips
Parallel bars
Pommel Horse
Vaulting Horse
Rowing Machine
Skipping Rope
Stepper
Trampoline

AU CENTRE
DE REMISE EN FORME
AU CENTRE DE BIEN-ÊTRE
AU GYMNASE

Quelles facilités sont disponibles au Centre de Remise en Forme?

Nous avons une piscine, le badminton, le tennis, un gymnase et le sauna
Vous pouvez choisir les cours ou les activités qui vous interesse
Les cours collectifs sont nombreux et très variés.
Je voudrais faire des cours de remise en forme.
Je voudrais faire un cours d'aquagym.
Quelles machines de exercice avez-vousdans le gymnase ?
Nous avons un grand choix de machines.
Vous pouvez réserver les équipments à la Reception.

Le Haltère Long
Le Extenseur
Le Haltère Court
Le Vélo d'Exercice
La Poignée à Ressort
Les Barres Parallèles
Le Cheval d'Arçons
Le Cheval-Sautoir
Le Rameur
La Corde à Sauter
Le Simulateur d'Escalier
La Trampoline

Treadmill	Le Tapis Motorisé / de Course
Twist Bar	Le Ressort Athlétique
Weight Trainer	Le Banc de Musculation

COLOURING YOUR HAIR AT HOME
SE TEINTE LES CHEVEUX CHEZ-SOI

Note: Hair Colouring Packs can be purchased at the chemist and the supermarket. Read the instructions before beginning.

Note: On peut acheter les produits de coloration à la pharmacie et au supermarché. Lisez les instructions avant de commencer.

PRODUCT SAFETY WARNINGS

PRÉCAUTIONS D'EMPLOI

Do Not Use If:
you have already experienced a reaction to a hair colourant or if you have sensitive, itchy or damaged scalp.
Consult your doctor for your individual sensitivity.
Perform a skin test 48 hours before using the product, even if you have used a hair colourant previously.

Ne Pas Utiliser Si:
vous avez déjà réagi à un produit de coloration vous avez le cuir chevelu sensible, irrité ou abîmé.
Consultez votre médecin à votre sensibilité personnelle.
Faire le test de sensibilité 48 heures avant l'utilisation de ce produit, même si vous avez déjà utilisé auparavant un produit de coloration.

In case of reaction during application,
rinse immediately in lukewarm water and consult your doctor.
Avoid contact with eyes.
Rinse eyes immediately if product comes into contact with them.
Take out contact lenses before rinsing well.

En cas de reaction pendant l'application, rincez immédiatement à l'eau tiède et consultez un médecin.
Éviter le contact du produit avec les yeux. Rincer immédiatement les yeux si le produit entre en contact avec ceux-ci. Si vous portez des lentilles de contact, retirez-les

Wear suitable gloves as supplied in the product carton.
Rinse hair well after application of the mixture.
Do not use the product to colour eyelashes and eyebrows, or any purpose other than colouring your hair.

Do not use on children.
Keep out of the reach of children.
If you have recently permed hair, normally wait 2 weeks before applying colour.

Never leave the colourant mixture on your hair for longer than recommended.

PACK CONTENTS

1 x pair of gloves (often attached to instruction leaflet)
1 x applicator bottle containing the Developer Milk
1 x tube of colour crème
1 x sachet of crème conditioner

APPLICATION

Put on gloves.
Unscrew applicator bottle containing the Developing Milk.
Pierce the colour crème tube and squeeze ALL the contents

avant de rincer vos yeux abondamment à l'eau
Porter les gants appropriés fournis dans l'étui.
Bien rincer les cheveux après application du mélange.
Ne pas employer pour la coloration des cils et des sourcils, ou pour un usage autre que la coloration des cheveux .

Ne pas utiliser chez enfant.
Ne pas laisser à la portée des enfants.
Si vos cheveux sont permanents, attendez 15 jours entre la permanente et la coloration.

Jamais laisser le produit longtemps, regardez les précautions d'emploi.

CONTENU D'ÉTUI

1 x paire de gants (souvent à décoller de le mode d'emploi)
1 x flacon applicateur contenant le lait révélateur
1 x tube de crème colorante
1 x sachet de crème bain

APPLICATION

Mettez les gants.
Dévissez le flacon applicateur contenant le lait révélateur.

Percez le tube de crème et versez la totalité dans le flacon

into the applicator bottle.	applicateur.
Firmly screw on the cap of the applicator bottle and shake thoroughly to an even mixture.	Rebouchez le flacon applicateur et agitez pour obtenir un mélange homogène.
Immediately break off the snap-off tip of the applicator bottle and apply product to hair as soon as possible:-	Cassez l'extrémité de l'embout applicateur immédiatement après mélange et procédez immédiatement à l'application:-
Protect your shoulders with an old towel. Wear the gloves provided. Apply to dry, unwashed hair, using the applicator bottle to guide the colour on to your hair.	Placez une serviette de protection sur vos épaules. Conservez les gants. Mettez application sur cheveux secs, non lavés, à l'aide du flacon applicateur.
If you have grey hair start at the temples or the roots.	Si vous avez des cheveux blancs, commencez par les zones tempes ou racines.
Massage product evenly through all of your hair, using all of the mixture.	Malaxez le produit et répartisez sur l'ensemble bien de la chevelure. Utilisez la totalité du mélange.
If you have little or no grey hair, leave to develop for (20)* minutes. For more than 70% grey hair, allow (30)* minutes.	Si vous avez peu ou pas de cheveux blancs, laissez agir (20)* minutes. Si vous avez beaucoup de cheveux blancs (+ 70%) laissez agir (30)* minutes.
* times may vary according to product – check leaflet. After development time, apply a little lukewarm water to the hair and massage gently. Rinse thoroughly until water runs clear.	* variable – vérifiez le mode d'emploi. Après le temps de pause, ajoutez un peu d'eau tiède et massez légèrement. Rincez ensuite abondamment jusqu'a ce que l'eau soit

Apply the entire contents of the crème conditioner and massage in to the hair.
Rinse thoroughly, until the water runs clear.
Dry and style as usual.

NEVER KEEP ANY UNUSED MIXTURE.
DISPOSE OF IT IMMEDIATELY.

claire.
Versez sur l'ensemble de la chevelure la totalité du bain crème et malaxez doucement.
Rincez abondamment jusqu'a ce que l'eau soit claire.
Coiffez-vous comme à votre habitude.
NE CONSERVEZ JAMAIS LE RESTE DU MÉLANGE
JETEZ-LE IMMÉDIATEMENT.

APPLYING A FACE PACK / MASK AT HOME
SE FAIRE UN MASQUE CHEZ-SOI

Note: Face Packs can be purchased at the chemist and at the supermarket.
Read the instructions before beginning
Warning:-
The product combines oils to deep cleanse whilst moisturizing.
Test sensitivity to natural oils – apply a small amount of neat product to inside of upper arm. Leave for 5 minutes. If reaction occurs, do not use.

For best effects :-
Thoroughly cleanse face
Apply product evenly over the face, avoiding eyes and lips.
Leave on for 10 – 15 minutes, then rinse off with water. Pat dry.
Leaves skin feeling smooth and radiant.

Note: On peut acheter les masques de beauté à la pharmacie et au supermarché
Lisez les instructions avant de commencer.
Attention:-
Ce produit associe de huiles pour nettoyer en profondeur tout en hydratant
Test de sensibilité aux huiles naturelles – appliquez une petite quantité de produit pur a l'interieur du bras. Attendez 5 minutes. En cas de reaction, ne pas utiliser le produit.

Pour un effet maximum :-
Bien nettoyer le visage.
Étaler ensuite la masque en evitant les yeux et la bouche
Laisser agir 10 – 15 minutes, puis rincer et secher.

Donne un peau douce et un teint radieux

ENGLISH-FRENCH DICTIONARY

A

abdomen; hypogastric region hypogastre *m*
above / below or under au-dessus / au-dessous *adv*
acne rosacea acné *f* rosacée
acupuncture; insertion of needles into skin acupuncture *f*
adorned hair style (special occasion style) gaufrage *m*
aerobics aérobic *m*
Afro afro *adj*
after-shave lotion; after-shave lotion *f* après-rasage; après-rasage *m*
after-shave; after-shave lotion lotion *f* after-shave
allergy, skin allergie *f* cutanée
alopecia alopecie *f*; pelade *f*
ankle cheville *f*
ankle joint articulation *f* de la cheville
anti-dandruff lotion lotion *f* contre les pellicules
anti-wrinkle cream crème *f* anti-rides
anti-wrinkle face-pack masque *m* anti-rides
antiseptic antiseptique *m*
application of products to eliminate toxins; wrappings enveloppements *mpl*
applicator bottle flacon *m* applicateur
apply blusher, to (to cheeks) rougir *v*
appointment rendez-vous *m*
arm bras *m*
armpit aisselle *f*
aromatherapy; essential oils massage and/or baths aromathérapie *f*
artificial hair cheveux *mpl* postiches
astringent lotion lotion *f* astringente
athlete's foot mycose *m* du pied
auburn (hair colour) auburn *adj, inv*; blond *m* ardent; blonde *f* ardente; cheveux *mpl* aux reflets cuivrés
auburn; titian (hair colour) châtain roux *adj*

B

back of the hand dos *m* de la main
backcomb, to; to tease crêper *v*
bald; hairless chauve *adj*
balding; receding dégarni,-e *adj*
baldness; bald patch: bald head calvitie *f* totale
ball of the foot eminence de l'articulation *f*
balneology; medically prescribed (21 day) cure thermalisme *m*
balneotherapy; bathing treatment balnéothérapie *f*
barber barbier *m*
barber maître-coiffeur *m*
barber shop salon *m* de coiffure pour hommes
bare nu,-e *adj*
barefoot nu-pieds *adj, adv*; (les) pieds nus
bareheaded nu-tête *adj, adv*; (la) tête nue
base of thumb joint eminence thénar *f*
basin / bowl cuvette *f*
bath bain *m*
- **mud bath** bain *m* de boue
- **steam bath** bain *m* de vapeur
- **whirlpool bath** jacuzzi; bain *m* bouillonnant

bath towel serviette *f* de bain
beard barbe *f*
- **full beard** barbe *f* longue
- **goatee beard** barbe *f* en pointe
- **small pointed beard** barbiche *f*
- **to have a beard** porter *v* la barbe
- **to shave off somebody's beard; to trim somebody's beard** faire la barbe à quelqu'un

beautician esthéticienne *f*
beauty beauté *f*
beauty care soins *mpl* esthétiques
beauty product produit *m* de beauté
beauty salon / parlour institut *m* de beauté
beauty spot; mole grain *m* de beauté
beauty treatment cure *f* de beauté
beauty treatment; beauty care soins *mpl* de beauté

birthmark   tache *f* de naissance
bite one's nails (to)   ronger (se) *v* les ongles
blackhead   point *m* noir
blade, razor   lame *f* de rasoir
bleach   agent *m* de décoloration
bleach (to)   décolorer *v*
bleach tube   tube *m* de produit décolorant
bleached hair   cheveux *mpl* décolorés ; cheveux *mpl* oygénés
bleaching   décoloration *f*
bleaching product   produit *m* décolorant
blond   blond, blonde adj
blond, blonde   blond *m*, blonde *f*
- **ash blonde; ash blond**   blond cendré *inv*
- **peroxide blonde**   blonde *f* oxygenée
- **platinum blonde**   blonde *f* platine

blond, to go; to bleach (hair)   blondir *v*
blow-dry   brushing *m*
- **to give somebody a blow-dry**   faire un brushing à quelqu'un
- **to have a blow-dry**   se faire faire un brushing

blue-rinsed hair   cheveux *mpl* aux reflets bleutés
blusher   fard *m* à joues
body   corps *m*
body care   soins *mpl* corporels; soins du corps; soins *mpl* de la peau
body hair   poil *m*
bottle blonde (not natural blond hair)   fausse blonde *f*
bottom (cheek) / buttock   fesse *f*
breast   sein *m*
brittle hair   cheveux *mpl* cassants
brittle nails   ongles *mpl* cassant
brown; brown-haired   châtain *adj*
brown; brownish   brunet, brunette *adj*
bruise; blue (colour)   bleu *m*
brunette   brunette *f*
brush (to) (hair etc)   brosser *v*
brush   brosse *f*
- **curling brush**   brosse *f* à boucler les cheveux
- **detangling brush**   brosse *f* à démêler les cheveux
- **hairbrush**   brosse *f* à cheveux
- **nail brush**   brosse *f* à ongles

- **round brush** brosse *f* ronde
- **warm air brush** brosse séche-cheveux *f*

bun; chignon; French pleat (hair style) chignon *m*
bunion oignon (pied) *m*

C

calf (of leg) mollet *m*
callus callosité *f*
callus; corn durillon *m*
cape; gown (at hairdresser's) peignoir *m*
care soin *m*; soins *mpl*
chair arm rest accoudoir *m*
chair arm rest bras *m* du fauteuil
chair footrest repose-pieds *m*
chair height adjuster bar la barre *f* de réglage (d'un fauteuil)
cheek (face) joue *f*
cheekbone pommette *f*
chest; breasts; bosom poitrine *f*
chilblain engelure *f*
chin menton *m*
chiropody; pedicure pédicurie *f*; podologie *f*
clean-shaven visage rasé *m*
clip (to) (hair) tondre *v*
clip or crop someone's hair (to) tondre *v* quelqu'un
clippers, electric clippers (hair) tondeuse *f* électrique
close-cropped (hair, head) ras, rase *adj*
close-cropped hair cheveux *mpl* coupés ras
coil (to) (hair) torsader *v*
coiled plaits diadème *m*
cold sore bouton *m* de fièvre
colour ; shade ; tint couleur *f*
colour brightener rinse dose *f* couleur
colour highlights (hair) mèches *fpl* de couleur
colour rinse (non-permanent) rinçage colorant *m*
colour stripping / removal décapage *v*
comb peigne *m*; peigne *m* de parure
- **Afro comb** peigne *m* afro; peigne africain

- **back comb; side comb** peigne *m* à chignon
- **dressing comb** démêloir *m*; gros peigne *m*
- **fine-tooth** (for headlice) peigne *m* à poux
- **finishing/dressing comb** peigne fin *m*
- **hair comb** peigne *m* de coiffure
- **hairdresser's comb; barber's comb** peigne *m* de coiffeur
- **large-toothed comb; dressing comb; rake comb (animal)** démêloir *m*
- **pocket comb** peigne *m* de poche
- **tail comb** peigne *m* à tige
- **teaser comb** peigne *m* à crêper
- **warm-air comb** peigne *m* soufflant ; peigne sèche-cheveux

comb, to (hair); **comb out, to** (hair) peigner *v*
comb one's hair (to) se peigner *v*
comb through one's hair (to run a) peigne m: se donner un coup de peigne
comb-out coup *m* de peigne
consultation room; surgery cabinet *m* de consultation
corn (on foot) cor *m*
cosmetic scrub (body / facial) gommage *m* (du corps / du visage)
cosmetic; beauty product; toiletry cosmétique *m*
course of hydrotherapy; water cure cure *f* thermale
course of thalassotherapy cure *f* de thalassothèrapie
course of treatment (eg at a spa) cure *f*
cream crème *f*
- **day cream** crème *f* de jour
- **face cream** crème *f* pour le visage
- **foundation cream** crème *f* de base
- **hand cream** crème *f* pour les mains
- **moisturizing cream** crème *f* hydratante
- **night cream** crème *f* de nuit
- **suntan cream** crème *f* solaire

crew cut; en brosse coupe *f* en brosse
crimping iron / tongs fer *m* à crêper les cheveux
crop the hair short or close, to couper *v* ras les cheveux
crown; top of head crâne *m*
curl; ringlet; tress; lock (of hair) boucle *f* (de cheveux)
curl, little curl; little ringlet frisette *f*
curl (to); curl loosely (to) boucler *v*
- **curl someone's hair (to); crimp (to)** friser *v*

- **to have curly hair** friser *v*
- **to curl one's hair** se friser *v*
- **to have one's hair curled** boucler: se faire boucler les cheveux

curler frisoir *m*
curling tongs fer *m* à onduler; fer *m* à friser
curly hair style coiffure *f* bouclée
curly hair; curly locks cheveux *mpl* bouclés
cut (to) (hair) couper *v*
cut (to); to have a haircut couper *v*: se faire couper les cheveux
cut and blow-dry coupe *f* et brushing
cut: have one's hair cut (to) couper *v*: se faire couper les cheveux
cuticle envie *f*; petites peaux *fpl*
cuticle pen; cuticle remover repousse-peaux *m*
cuticle remover crème *f* émolliente

D

dandruff pellicules *fpl*
dark (in colour) sombre *adj*
dark / light brown hair cheveux *mpl* châtain foncé / clair
deodorant stick stick *m* : déodorant en stick
depilatory dépilatoire *m*
detangle (to) démêler *v*
detox (to) désintoxiquer *v*
detoxification cure *f* de désintoxication
diabetic diabétique f; also *adj*
diet régime *m*
diet, fat/salt/sugar-free diet régime *m* sans graisse/sel/sucre
dimple fossette *f* mentonnière; fossette au menton
disposable razor rasoir *m* jetable
dizziness vertiges *mpl*
dose; measure; amount dose *f*
dreadlocks dreadlocks *fpl*
dry out (to) dessécher *v*
dry shampoo shampooing sec *m*
dye one's hair se teindre *v*

E

ear orielle *f*
ear lobe lobe *m* de l'oreille
earring boucle *f* d'oreille
• **drop earring** pendant d'orielle *f*
effleurage; light massage effleurage *m*
electrolysis électrolyse *f*
essential oils huiles essentielles *f*
exercise exercice *m*
exercise bicycle vélo *m* d'entraînement; vélo d'appartement
exercise programme programme *m* d'exercices
exfoliating scrub exfoliant *m*
eye œil *m*
eye-shadow fard *m* à paupières
eye socket orbite *f*
eyebrow sourcil *m*
eyebrow pencil crayon *m* à sourcils
eyedrops gouttes (pour les yeux) *fpl*
eyelash cil; cilium *m*
eyelashes, false; artificial eyelashes cils *mpl* faux
eyelid lower paupière *f* inferieure
eyelid upper paupière *f* supérieure
eyeliner pencil crayon *m* pour les yeux

F

face visage *m*
face lift lifting *m* ; déridage *m*
face pack masque *m* de beauté
face powder; rice powder poudre *f* de riz
facial soin *m* (complet) du visage
facial hair poils *mpl* du visage
fairness; blondness blondeur *f*; couleur *f* blonde
fever fièvre *f*
fine fine *adj*

finger little doigt *m*: auriculaire *m*
finger middle doigt *m*: majeur *m*
finger nail ongle *m*
finger pad pulpe *f* de la phalangette
finger tip bout *m* du doigt
finger, ring; third finger doigt *m* annulaire
finger, index doigt *m* : index *m*
firm up, to; to tone up raffermir *v*
flaxen blond,-e *adj*
foot pied *m*
foot stool tabouret *m*
forehead front *m*
foundation; make-up base fond *m* de teint
freckle tache *f* de rousseur / tache de son (familiar)
fringe frange *f*
frizz (hair), to; to make curly frisotter / faire friser *v*
frizzy (hair) crépu / crêpelé *adj*
frizzy hair cheveux *mpl* crépés

G

glasses; spectacles lunettes *fpl*
golden doré,-e *adj* (eg hair)
golden-haired cheveux *mpl* dorés
greying; grey-haired grisonnant,-e; aux cheveux gris *adj*
grow a beard, to se laisser pousser *v* la barbe
gymnasium gymnase *m*

H

hair cheveux *mpl*
hair colouring; hair tinting coloration *f* des cheveux
hair conditioner démêlant *m* ; baume *m* démêlant; après-shampooing *m*
hair cream crème *f* coiffante
hair crimper fer *m* à gaufrer
hair cropped close cheveux *mpl* coupés ras
hair curler / roller rouleau *m* (à mise en plis)

hair curling clip pince *f* à boucle de cheveux
hair cut; hair style coupe *f* de cheveux
hair drying (finger dry) séchage *m* rapide
hair extensions extensions *fpl*
hair follicle follicule *m* pileux
hair gel gel *m* coiffant
hair lacquer; hairspray laque *m* pour cheveux
hair lotion; hair tonic lotion *f* capillaire; lotion revitalisante
hair mousse mousse *f* coiffante
hair net filet à cheveux *m*; résille *f*
hair piece postiche *m* de cheveux
hair regrowth repousse *f* de cheveux
hair removing cream crème *f* dépilatoire
hair restorer régénérateur *m* des cheveux
hair roller (setting roller) rouleau *m* (à mise en plis)
hair set (strong) mise *f* en plis (soutien)
hair setting lotion lotion *f* coiffante
hair straightener défrisant *m*
hair style; hairdo coiffure *f*
hair tonic; toning lotion tonique *m*
hair transplant / graft greffe *f* de cheveu
hair, brown cheveux *mpl* bruns
hair, difficult hair cheveux *mpl* à problèmes
hair, fair hair; blond hair cheveux *mpl* blonds
hair, well-cared for hair cheveux *mpl* soignés
hair, white hair cheveux *mpl* blancs
hair-oil huile *f* capillaire
hair: give one's hair body (to) donner *v* du volume à ses cheveux
hair: give your hair bounce (to) pour donner du volume à vos cheveux
hair; tresses chevelure *f*
hairband; headband; fillet; alice-band; circlet bandeau *m*; serre-tête *m*
haircare soins *mpl* de cheveu
hairclip pince *f* (à cheveux)
hairclip; hair slide barrette *f*
haircut (to have a) tailler *v* : se faire tailler les cheveux
haircut; hair-cutting taille *f* de cheveux
hairdresser coiffeuse *f*
hairdresser / barber coiffeur *m* ; le maître-coiffeur
hairdresser's tools ustensiles *mpl* de coiffure

hairdressing salon salon *m* de coiffure pour dames
hairdrier (eg fixed drier at hairdresser) casque *m* de séchage
hairdrier socket prise *f* (de sèche-cheveux)
hairdrier; salon swivel dryer séchoir *m*
hairless; bare (of face) nu, nue *adj*
hairline naissance *f* des cheveux
hairnet filet *m* à cheveux; résille *f*
hairpiece fausse mèche *f*
hairpin épingle *f* à cheveux
hairspray; lacquer fixatif *m*
hand main *f*
hand drier sèche-cheveux *m*
hand mirror miroir *m* à main
hangnail envie *f*; filet *m* de peau
head-rest (on barber's chair) appui-tête *m*
health food shop magasin *m* de produits diététiques
heel of foot talon *m*
henna henné *m*
henna (to) (hair) teindre *v* au henné
highlight; streak (in hair); lock (of hair) mèche *f*
highlights put in hair, (to have); to have one's hair streaked (eg blond)
  mèche *f*: se faire faire des mèches ; se faire faire un balayage
hip hanche *f*
hot flush bouffée *f* de chaleur
hurt, to blesser *v* ; faire du mal à

IJK

implant implant *m*
instep cou-de-pied *m*
iris of the eye iris *m*
itch (to) démanger *v*
jacuzzi; whirlpool bath jacuzzi *m*
jaw mâchoire *f*
jogging jogging *m*
keratin kératine *f*
knee genou *m*
knuckle articulation *f* ; jointure *f* du doigt

L

lank (hair); dull (hair) raide et terne *adj*
lanolin lanoline *f*
layer (in hair); layered cut dégradé *m*
layered cut coupe *f* dégradée
leg jambe *f*
lightening (of hair) éclaircissante *adj*
lip lèvre *f*
lip gloss brillant *m* à lèvres
lip liner pencil crayon *m* à lèvres
lip salve pommade *f* rosat; pommade *f* pour les lèvres
lip, lower lèvre *f* inférieure
lip, upper lèvre *f* supérieure
liposuction liposuccion *f*
lipstick rouge à lèvres *m*
lipstick; lipstick case bâton *m* de rouge à lèvres ; tube *m* de rouge à lèvres
lotion, body lait *m* pour le corps
lotion: setting lotion spray can atomiseur *m* de fixative pour cheveux
louse; lice *(pl)* pou m; poux mpl

M

make-up bag / purse trousse *f* de maquillage
make-up gown serviette *f* de maquillage
make-up remover démaquillant *m*
make-up table table de maquillage *f*
make-up; making-up maquillage *m*
manicure soin *m* des mains
manicure set; manicure case trousse *f* de manucure; trousse à ongles
manicure; manicurist manucure *f*
mascara mascara *m*
massage massage *m*
massage for elimination of dead skin cells exfoliation *f* (see also gommage)
massage parlour institut de massage *m*

masseur; masseuse masseur *m*; masseuse *f*
melanin mélanine *f*
mix, to malaxer *v*
mixer tap mélangeur *m* ; mitigeur *m* ; robinet *m* mélangeur
mixing malaxage *m*
moustache, military style; moustache, toothbrush style moustache *f* en brosse
moustache, short moustache *f* courte
moustache, walrus moustache *f* à la gauloise
mouth bouche *f*
mouthwash bain *m* de bouche
mud boue *f*

N

nail cleaner; orange stick cure-ongles *m inv*
nail clippers pince *f* à ongles
nail crescent lunule *f*
nail file; emery board lime *f* à ongles
nail varnish vernis *m* à ongles
nail varnish remover dissolvant *m*
nape of the neck nuque *f*
neck cou *m*
needle aiguille *f*
nose nez *m*
nose stud anneau *m* de nez
nostril hair vibrisse *f*
nutritive cream treatment for coloured / permed hair soins *mpl* protection (couleur / perm)

P

package, inclusive (eg for spa treatment) forfait *m*
pageboy style coiffure *f* à frange
palm of hand paume *f*
paper collar-towel col *m* de papier *m*

part one's hair on the right/ left/ in the middle (to) raie *f*: porter la raie à droite/ à gauche/ au milieu
parting (of hair) raie *f*
pedicure, to have a pied: se faire soigner les pieds *f*
perfume; scent; flavour parfum *m*
perm; permanent wave (hair) permanente *f*
permanent: to have a perm permanente *f*: se faire faire une permanente
peroxide peroxyde *m*
person taking the waters at a spa curiste *m/f*
perspiration /sweat sueur *f*
perspiration; sweat; perspiring transpiration *f*
petrissage; kneading massage petrissage *m*
pierce, to; to have pierced (eg ears) percer (se faire) *v*
pierced ears oreilles *fpl* percées
piercing (eg of body, ears) perçant, perçante *adj*
pimple; spot bouton *m*
plait tresse *f*
plait (to); to braid tresser *v*; natter *v*
plaiting; braiding (US) tressage *m*
plaits; bunches (hairstyle) nattes *fpl*
plaster; dressing pansement *m*
plastic surgery chirurgie *f* plastique
pluck one's eyebrows, to épiler *v* : s'épiler les sourcils
pomade; pomatum pommade *f*
ponytail queue *f* de cheval
ponytail; pigtail; bow; hair ribbon cadogan *m*; catogan *m*
pot of cream pot *m* de crème
powder compact poudrier *m*
pregnant enceinte *adj*
preparation stage for colouring hair précoloration *f*
pubic area pubis *m*
pupil of the eye pupille *f*
put one's hair up, to relever *v* ses cheveux
put, to; to put on mettre *v*

R

range (of products/treatments) gamme *m*

razor rasoir *m*
razor, electric; electric shaver rasoir *m* électrique
razor, safety rasoir *m* de sûreté ; rasoir *m* mécanique; rasoir *m* américain
razor, thinning rasoir *m* à désépaissir; rasoir *m* effileur
re-style (to) changer *v* de coiffure
red-hair; redhead cheveux *m* roux
red-haired rouquin, rouquine *adj*
red-haired person; redhead rouquin *m*; rouquine *f*
reflexology; pressure on reflex areas of feet or hands réflexologie *f*
refreshed, to feel se sentir *v* revigoré
rejuvenating rajeunissant,-e *adj*
rejuvenation treatment cure *f* de jouvence
relax (to); release tension (to) détendre *v*
relax (to) relâcher *v*; relaxer *v*
removal of hair by waxing èpilation *f* à la cire
removal of superfluous hair épilation *f*; dépilation *f*
remove (to); take off (to) enlever *v*
remove hair from the legs (to); wax the legs (to) épiler *v* des jambes
revitalising revitalisantes *adj*
roots racines *fpl*
roots colour touch-up touching *v*

S

salon chair, adjustable fauteuil *m* réglable
sauna sauna *m*
scab croûte *f*
scalp cuir *m* chevelu
scar cicatrice *f*
scissors, cutting ciseaux *mpl* de coupe
scissors, hairdressing ciseaux *mpl* de coiffeur
scissors, manicure ciseaux *mpl* de manucure / à ongles
scissors, thinning ciseaux *mpl* à effiler (à désépaissir)
screen (for electric razor) grille *f* (pour rasoir electrique)
sea water treatment thalassothérapie *f*
semi-permanent colour couleur *f* temporaire
serum serum *m*
shampoo shampooing *m*

- **herbal shampoo** shampooing *m* herbal ou aux herbes
- **medicated shampoo treatment** shampooing *m* traitant
- **soft; gentle acting shampoo** shampooing *m* doux

shampoo, to shampouiner *v*
shampoo and cut shampooing *m* et coupe *f*
shampoo and set shampooing *m* et mise en plis
shampoo bottle bouteille *f* de shampooing
shampoo one's hair (to) shampooing: se faire un shampooing
shampoo someone's hair (to) shampooing *m*: faire ou donner un shampooing à quelqu'un
shampooed (to have one's hair) shampooing *m* : se faire faire un shampooing
shampooer (person) shampouineur *m*; shampouineuse *f*
shaping up remise en forme *v*
shave (to); to have a shave se raser *v*
shave (to); to shave off raser *v*
shave one's head (to) se raser *v* la tête
shaved (to get); to have a shave; to get a shave se raser; se faire raser
shaved, to shave one's head se faire raser *v* la tête
shaving (of beard) rasage *m*
shaving brush blaireau *m*
shaving cream crème *f* à raser
shaving stick stick à raser *m*
shiatsu; Japanese needleless acupuncture massage method shiatsu *n*
shingle; bobbed hair style coiffure *f* à la garçonne
shoes chaussures *fpl*
short haircut; bob coiffure *f* courte
short-back-and-sides coupe *f* classique - homme
shoulder épaule *f*
show, to montrer *v*
shower spray on wash basin douche *f* à main
sideburn; sideboard; side-of-face hair patte *f*
sideburns; whiskers (out-dated) favoris *mpl*
size; waist; waistline taille *f*
skin (greasy / dry / sensitive) peau *f* (grasse / sèche / sensible)
skin blemish abîmé *f*
skin boil; furuncle furoncle *m*
skin graft greffe *f* de peau
skin test cuti-réaction *f*

skincare soins *mpl* de la peau
sleep therapy cure *f* de sommeil
slim mince *adj*
slim, to; slimmer, to get amincer (s') *v*
slim, to; to lose weight maigrir *v*
slimming amincissant,-e *adj*
slimming course cure *f* d'amaigrissement
small-tooth comb peigne *m* fin
soap savon *m*
soap dish porte-savon *m*
socks chaussettes *fpl*
solarium solarium *m*
sole of the foot plante *f* du pied
solution (chemical; pharmaceutical) soluté *m*
spa station *f* thermale
spine colonne *f* vertébrale
split ends fourches *fpl*
spot / pimple tache *f*
spray can (hair / deodorant) bombe *f* (pour cheveux / déodorante)
spray; atomiser; facial mister brumisateur *m*
stones on body's energy points stonethérapie *f*
straight hair cheveux *mpl* raides
straighten (to) (hair) défriser *v*
stray lock méche *f* folle
stubble barbe *f* de trois jours
stud earring boucle *f* d'oreille
sun block crème *f* écran total
sunbathe, (to) bronzer: se faire bronzer
sunbathe, to se dorer au soleil
sunburn coup *m* de soleil
sunglasses lunettes *fpl* de soleil
sunlamp lampe *f* à bronzer
sunscreen écran *m* solaire
suntan lotion lotion *f* solaire
suntan lotion factor 8 crème *f* solaire facteur 8
swimming pool piscine *f*
switch postiche *m*

T

tan bronzage *m*
tan (to); to get a tan bronzer *v*
tap (hot / cold) robinet *m* d'eau chaude / froide
tattoo; tattooing tatouage *m*
temple (head) tempe *f*
thermal thermal,-e *adj*
thick épaisse *adj*
thigh cuisse *f*
thin out (to) (hair) désépaissir *v* (à main)
thinning out of hair (by hairdresser) éclaircissage *m*
throat gorge *f*
thumb pouce *m*
tickle (to) chatouiller *v*
ticklish chatouilleux, chatouilleuse *adj*
tinea; scalp disease teigne *f*
tint: to have one's hair tinted se faire faire une coloration
tinted hair; coloured hair cheveux *mpl* colorés
tip (money) pourboire *m*
toe nail ongle *m* de l'orteil
toe, big orteil *m* gros
toe, fourth orteil *m* quatrième
toe, little orteil *m* petit
toe, second orteil *m* deuxième
toe, third orteil *m* troisième
toilet water, perfumed; eau de Cologne eau *f* de toilette / eau de Cologne
top / crown of head sommet de la tête *m* (see crâne)
touch /massage lightly (to) effleurer *v*
towel serviette *f* (de toilette)
towel for drying hair serviette *f* de toilette pour sécher
towel for face compresses serviette *f* pour compresses / faciales
treatment traitement *m*
trim (3 or 4 cm) coupe *f* entretien
 • **to have a trim** se faire rafraîchir les cheveux
trim, to (the beard) faire *v* la barbe
trimmer (on electric razor) tondeuse *f*

tube of cream tube *m* de crème
turn golden, to dorer *v*
tweezers, eyebrow tweezers pince *f* à épiler

UW

undress, to déshabiller *v*
wall mirror miroir *m* mural
warm sea mud wrap fangothérapie *f*
wash basin lavabo *m*
wash in peroxide, to; to bleach oxygéner *v*
wave (to) (hair) onduler *v*
wavy hair cheveux *mpl* ondulés
wayward lock méche *f* rebelle
weight poids *m*
well-being bien-être *m*
wig; hairpiece perruque *f*
wig; hairpiece; piece of false hair postiche *m*
wig; hairpiece; toupee postiche *m*
wipe, to essuyer *v*
wrappings; application of products to eliminate toxins enveloppements *mpl*
wrinkle ride *f*
wrist poignet *m*

DICTIONARY FRENCH-ENGLISH

A

abîmé *f* skin blemish
accoudoir *m* chair arm rest
acné *f* **rosacée** acne rosacea
acuponcture *f* acupuncture; insertion of needles into skin

aérobic *m*   aerobics
afro *adj*   Afro
agent *m* **de décoloration**   bleach
aiguille *f*   needle
aisselle *f*   armpit
allergie *f* **cutanée**   allergy, skin
amincer (s') *v*   to slim; to get slimmer
amincissant,-e *adj*   slimming
anneau *m* **de nez**   nose stud
antiseptique *m*   antiseptic
appui-tête *m*   head rest (on barber's chair)
après-shampooing *m*   hair conditioner
aromathérapie *f*   aromatherapy; essential oils massage and/or baths
articulation f; œil *m* **de l'articulation; jointure** *f* **du doigt**   knuckle
atomiseur *m* **de fixative pour cheveux**   setting lotion spray can
au-dessus / au-dessous   *adv*   above / below or under
auburn *adj   inv*   auburn (hair colour)

B

bain *m* **bouillonnant**   whirlpool bath; jacuzzi
bain *m* **de bouche**   mouthwash
bain *m* **de boue**   mud bath
bain *m* **de vapeur**   steam bath
balayage *m*: **se faire faire un balayage**   to have highlights put in (hair)
balnéothérapie *f*   balneotherapy; bathing treatment (eg for arthritis)
bandeau *m*   hairband; headband; fillet; alice-band; circlet
barbe *f*   beard
- **faire la barbe**   to trim (the beard)
- **faire la barbe à quelqu'un**   to shave off somebody's beard; to trim somebody's beard
- **porter** *v* **la barbe**   to have a beard

barbe *f* **longue**   full beard
barbe *f* **de trois jours**   stubble
barbe *f* **en pointe**   goatee beard
barbiche *f*   goatee beard; small pointed beard
barbier *m*   barber
barrette *f*   hairclip; hair slide

baume *m* **démêlant**   hair conditioner
beauté *f*   beauty
bien-être *m*   well-being
bigoudi *m*   hair roller; hair curler
blaireau *m*   shaving brush
blesser *v*; **faire du mal à**   to hurt
bleu *m*   bruise; blue (colour)
blond,-e *adj*   flaxen
blond *m* **ardent; blonde** *f* **ardente**   auburn (hair clour)
blond cendré *inv*   ash blonde; ash blond
blonde *f* **oxygenée**   peroxide blonde
blondeur f; couleur *f* **blonde**   fairness; blondness
blondir *v*   to go blond; to bleach (hair)
bombe *f* **(pour cheveux / déodorante)**   spray can (hair / deodorant)
bouche *f*   mouth
boucle *f* **d'orielle**   earring; stud earring
boucle *f* **(de cheveux)**   curl; ringlet; tress ;lock (of hair)
boucler *v*   to curl; to curl loosely
  • **se faire boucler les cheveux**   to have one's hair curled
boue *f*   mud
bouffée *f* **de chaleur**   hot flush
bout *m* **du doigt**   finger tip
bouteille *f* **de shampooing**   shampoo bottle
bouton *m*   pimple; spot
bouton *m* **de fièvre**   cold sore
bras *m*   arm
bras *m* **du fauteuil**   chair arm rest
brillant *m* **à lèvres**   lip gloss
bronzage *m*   tan
bronzer *v*   to tan; to get a tan
  • **se faire bronzer**   to sunbathe
brosse *f* **ronde**   round brush
brosse *f* **à cheveux**   hairbrush
brosse *f* **à boucler les cheveux**   curling brush
brosse *f* **à démêler les cheveux**   detangling brush
brosse *f* **à ongles**   nail brush
brosse *f* **séche-cheveux**   warm air brush
brosser *v*   to brush (hair etc)
brumisateur *m*   spray; atomiser; facial mister

brunet, brunette *adj* brown; brownish
brunette *f* brunette
brushing *m* blow-dry
• **faire un brushing à quelqu'un** to give somebody a blow-dry
• **se faire faire un brushing** to have a blow-dry

C

cabinet *m* **de consultation** consultation room; surgery
cadogan m; catogan *m* ponytail; pigtail; bow; hair ribbon
callosité *f* callus
calvitie *f* **totale** baldness; bald patch: bald head
casque *m* **de séchage** hairdrier (eg fixed drier at hairdresser)
châtain *adj* brown; brown-haired
châtain roux *adj* auburn ; titian (hair colour)
chatouiller *v* tickle (to)
chatouilleux, chatouilleuse *adj* ticklish
chaussettes *fpl* socks
chaussures *fpl* shoes
chauve *adj* bald; hairless
chevelure *f* hair; tresses
cheveux *mpl* hair
cheveux *mpl* **à problèmes** difficult hair
cheveux *mpl* **aux reflets bleutés** blue-rinsed hair
cheveux *mpl* **aux reflets cuivrés** auburn (hair clour)
cheveux *mpl* **blancs** white hair
cheveux *mpl* **blonds** fair hair; blond hair
cheveux *mpl* **bouclés** curly hair; curly locks
cheveux *mpl* **bruns** brown hair
cheveux *mpl* **cassants** brittle hair
cheveux *mpl* **châtain foncé / clair** dark / light brown hair
cheveux *mpl* **colorés** tinted hair; coloured hair
cheveux *mpl* **coupés ras** close-cropped hair ; hair cropped close
cheveux *mpl* **crêpés** frizzy hair
cheveux *mpl* **décolorés** bleached hair
• **donner** *v* **du volume à ses cheveux** to give one's hair body
cheveux *mpl* **ondulés** wavy hair
cheveux *mpl* **oygénés** bleached hair

cheveux *mpl* **postiches**   artificial hair
cheveux *mpl* **raides**   straight hair
cheveux *mpl* **soignés**   well-cared for hair
cheville *f*   ankle
chignon *m*   bun; chignon; French pleat (hair style)
chirurgie *f* **plastique**   plastic surgery
cicatrice *f*   scar
cil; cilium *m*   eyelash
cils *mpl* **faux**   false eyelashes; artificial eyelashes
ciseaux *mpl* **de coiffeur**   hairdressing scissors
ciseaux *mpl* **de coupe**   cutting scissors
ciseaux *mpl* **à effiler (à désépaissir)** *m*   thinning scissors
ciseaux *mpl* **de manucure / à ongles**   manicure scissors
coiffeur *m*; **le maître-coiffeur**   hairdresser / barber
coiffeuse *f*   hairdresser
coiffure *f*   hair style; hairdo
coiffure *f* **à frange**   pageboy style
coiffure *f* **à la garçonne**   shingle; bobbed hair style
coiffure *f* **bouclée**   curly hair style
coiffure *f* **courte**   short haircut; bob
col *m* **de papier** *m*   paper collar-towel
colonne *f* **vertébrale**   spine
coloration *f* **des cheveux**   hair colouring; hair tinting
  • **se faire faire une coloration**   to have one's hair tinted
cor *m*   corn (on foot)
corps *m*   body
cosmétique *m*   cosmetic; beauty product; toiletry
cou *m*   neck
cou-de-pied *m*   instep; ankle joint
couleur *f*   colour, shade, tint
coup *m* **de soleil**   sunburn
coupe *f* **classique - homme**   short-back-and-sides
coupe *f* **de cheveux**   hair cut; hair style
coupe *f* **dégradée**   layered cut
coupe *f* **en brosse**   crew cut; en brosse
coupe *f* **entretien**   trim (3 or 4 cm off hair)
coupe *f* **et brushing**   cut and blow-dry
couper *v*   to cut (hair)
  • **se faire couper les cheveux**   to have one's hair cut; to have a haircut

crâne *m* crown; top of head
crayon *m* **à lèvres** lip liner pencil
crayon *m* **à sourcils** eyebrow pencil
crayon *m* **pour les yeux** eyeliner pencil
crème *f* cream
crème *f* **à raser** shaving cream
crème *f* **anti-rides** anti-wrinkle cream
crème *f* **coiffante** hair cream
crème *f* **de base** foundation cream
crème *f* **de jour** day cream
crème *f* **de nuit** night cream
crème *f* **dépilatoire** hair removing cream
crème *f* **écran** total sun block
crème *f* **émolliente** cuticle remover
crème *f* **hydratante** moisturizing cream
crème *f* **pour le visage** face cream
crème *f* **pour les mains** hand cream
crème *f* **solaire** suntan cream
crème *f* **solaire facteur 8** suntan lotion factor 8
crêper *v* to backcomb ; to tease
crépu / crêpelé *adj* frizzy (hair)
croûte *f* scab
cuir *m* **chevelu** scalp
cuisse *f* thigh
cure *f* course of treatment (eg at a spa)
cure *f* **d'amaigrissement** slimming course
cure *f* **de beauté** beauty treatment
cure *f* **de thalassothèrapie** course of thalassotherapy
cure *f* **de désintoxication** detoxification
cure *f* **de jouvence** rejuvenation treatment
cure *f* **de sommeil** sleep therapy
cure *f* **thermale** course of hydrotherapy; water cure
cure-ongles *m inv* nail cleaner; orange stick
curiste *m/f* person taking the waters at a spa
cuti-réaction *f* skin test
cuticule *f* cuticle
cuvette *f* basin / bowl

D

décapage *v*   colour stripping / removal
décoloration *f*   bleaching
décolorer *v*   bleach (to)
défrisant *m*   hair straightener
défriser *v*   to straighten (hair)
dégarni,-e *adj*   balding; receding
dégradé *m*   layer (in hair); layered cut
démanger *v*   to itch
démaquillant *m*   make-up remover
démelant *m*   hair conditioner
démêler *v*   to detangle
démêloir *m*   large-toothed comb; dressing comb; rake comb (animal)
dépilatoire *m*   depilatory
déridage *m*   face lift
désépaissir *v* **(à main)**   to thin out (hair)
déshabiller *v*   to undress
désintoxiquer *v*   to detox
dessécher *v*   to dry out
détendre *v*   to relax; to release tension
diabétique *f*; also *adj*   diabetic
diadème *m*   coiled plaits
diète *f*   diet
dissolvant *m*   nail varnish remover
doigt *m* **annulaire**   ring finger; third finger
doigt *m*: **auriculaire** *m*   little finger
doigt *m* : **index** *m*   index finger
doigt *m*:**majeur** *m*   middle finger
dorer *v*   to turn golden
dorer (se) au soleil   to sunbathe
  • **cheveux** *mpl* **dorés**   golden hair; golden-haired
dos *m* **de la main**   back of the hand
dose *f*   dose; measure; amount
dose *f* **couleur**   colour brightener rinse
douche *f* **à main**   shampoo spray on wash basin
dreadlocks *fpl*   dreadlocks

durillon *m*   callus; corn

E

eau *f* **de toilette / eau de Cologne**   toilet water, perfumed; eau de Cologne
éclaircissage *m*   thinning out of hair (by hairdresser)
éclaircissante *adj*   lightening of hair
écran solaire *m*   sunscreen
effleurage *m*   effleurage; light massage
effleurer *v*   to touch /massage lightly
électrolyse *f*   electrolysis
eminence de l'articulation *f*   ball of the foot
eminence thénar *f*   base of thumb joint
enceinte *adj*   pregnant
engelure *f*   chilblain
enlever *v*   to remove; to take off
enveloppements *mpl*   application of products to eliminate toxins; wrappings
envie *f*; **petites peaux** *fpl*   cuticle
épaisse *adj*   thick
épaule *f*   shoulder
épilation *f*; **dépilation** *f*   removal of superfluous hair
èpilation *f* **à la cire**   removal of hair by waxing
épiler *v* **des jambes**   to remove hair from the legs; to wax the legs
pince *f* **à épiler**   eyebrow tweezers
épiler *v* : **s'épiler les sourcils**   to pluck one's eyebrows
épingle *f* **à cheveux**   hairpin
essuyer *v*   to wipe
esthéticienne *f*   beautician
exfoliation *f*   massage for elimination of dead skin cells
extensions *fpl* hair extensions

F

fangothérapie *f*   warm sea mud wrap
fard *m* **à joues**   blusher
fard *m* **à paupières**   eye-shadow

fausse blonde *f*   bottle blonde (not natural blonde hair)
fausse mèche *f*   hairpiece
fauteuil: la barre *f* **/ l'arceau** *m* **de réglage**   chair height adjuster bar
fauteuil *m* **réglable**   adjustable salon chair
favoris *mpl*   sideburns; whiskers (out-dated)
fer *m* **à crêper les cheveux**   crimping iron / tongs
fer *m* **à friser**   curling tongs / iron
fer *m* **à gaufrer**   hair crimper
fer *m* **à onduler**   curling tongs
fesse *f*   bottom (cheek) / buttock
fièvre *f*   fever
filet *m* **à cheveux**   hairnet
filet *m* **de peau ; envie** *f*   hangnail
fine *adj*   fine
fixatif *m*   hairspray; lacquer
flacon *m* **applicateur**   applicator bottle
follicule *m* **pileux**   hair follicle
fond *m* **de teint**   foundation; make-up base
forfait *m*   (inclusive) package
fossette *f* **mentonnière; fossette au menton**   dimple
fourches *fpl*   split ends
frange *f*   fringe
friser *v*   to curl; to have curly hair; to curl someone's hair; to crimp
friser (se) *v*   to curl one's hair
frisette *f*   little curl; little ringlet
frisoir *m*   curler
frisotter / faire friser *v*   to frizz (hair); to make curly
front *m*   forehead
furoncle *m*   skin boil; furuncle

G

gamme *m*   range (of products/treatments)
gaufrage *m*   adorned hair style (special occasion style)
gel *m* **coiffant**   hair gel
genou *m*   knee
gommage *m* **(du corps / du visage)**   cosmetic scrub (body / facial)
gorge *f*   throat

gouttes (pour les yeux) *fpl*   eyedrops
grain *m* **de beauté**   beauty spot; mole
greffe *f* **de cheveu**   hair transplant / graft
greffe *f* **de peau**   skin graft
grille *f* **(pour rasoir electrique)**   screen (for electric razor)
grisonnant,-e; aux cheveux gris *adj*   greying; grey-haired
gros peigne *m*   dressing comb
gymnase *m*   gymnasium

H

hanche *f*   hip
teindre *v* **au henné**   henna to (hair)
henné *m*   henna
huile *f* **capillaire**   hair-oil
huiles essentielles *f*   essential oils
hypogastre *m*   abdomen; hypogastric region

IJK

implant *m*   implant
institut *m* **de beauté**   beauty salon / parlour
institut de massage *m*   massage parlour
iris *m*   iris of the eye
jacuzzi *m*   jacuzzi; whirlpool bath
jambe *f*   leg
jogging *m*   jogging
joue *f*   cheek (face)
kératine *f*   keratin

L

lait *m* **pour le corps**   lotion, body lotion
lame *f* **de rasoir**   razor blade
lampe *f* **à bronzer**   sunlamp

lanoline *f*   lanolin
laque *m* **pour cheveux**   hair lacquer; hairspray
lavabo *m*   wash basin
lèvre *f*   lip
lèvre *f* **inférieure**   lower lip
lèvre *f* **supérieure**   upper lip
lifting *m*   face-lift
lime *f* **à ongles**   nail file; emery board
liposuccion *f*   liposuction
lobe *m* **de l'oreille**   ear lobe
lotion *f* **coiffante**   hair setting lotion
lotion *f* **after-shave**   after-shave; after-shave lotion
lotion *f* **après-rasage; après-rasage** *m*   after-shave lotion; after-shave
lotion *f* **astringente**   astringent lotion
lotion *f* **capillaire; lotion revitalisante**   hair lotion; hair tonic
lotion *f* **solaire**   suntan lotion
lunettes *fpl*   glasses; spectacles
lunettes *fpl* **de soleil**   sunglasses
lunule *f*   nail crescent

M

mâchoire *f*   jaw
maigrir *v*   to slim; to lose weight
main *f*   hand
maître-coiffeur *m*   barber
malaxage *m*   mixing
malaxer *v*   to mix
manucure *f*   manicure; manicurist
maquillage *m*   make-up; making-up
mascara *m*   mascara
masque *m* **de beauté**   face pack
masque *m* **antirides**   anti-wrinkle face-pack
massage *m*   massage
masseur *m*; **masseuse** *f*   masseur; masseuse
mèche *f*   highlight; streak (in hair); lock (of hair)
   • **se faire faire des mèches**   to have highlights put in hair; to have one's hair streaked (eg blond)

méche *f* **folle** stray lock
méche *f* **rebelle** wayward lock
mèches *fpl* **de couleur** colour highlights (hair)
mélangeur *m* mixer tap
mélanine *f* melanin
menton *m* chin
mettre *v* to put; to put on
mince *adj* slim
miroir *m* **à main** hand mirror
miroir *m* **mural** wall mirror
mise *f* **en plis (soutien)** hair set (strong)
mitigeur *m* mixer tap
mollet *m* calf (of leg)
montrer *v* to show
mousse *f* **coiffante** hair mousse
moustache *f* **courte** short moustache
moustache *f* **à la gauloise** walrus moustache
moustache *f* **en brosse** military style moustache; toothbrush style moustache
mycose *m* **du pied** athlete's foot

N

naissance *f* **des cheveux** hairline
natter *v* to plait; to braid
nattes *fpl* plaits; bunches (hairstyle)
nez *m* nose
nu, nue *adj* hairless; bare (of face)
nu-pieds *adj, adv*; **(les) pieds nus** barefoot
nu-tête *adj, adv*; **tête nu** *adj, adv* bareheaded
nuque *f* nape of the neck

O

œil *m* eye
oignon (pied) *m* bunion
onduler *v* to wave (hair)

ongle *m* finger nail
ongle de l'orteil *m* toe nail
ongles *mpl* **cassant** brittle nails
orbite *f* eye socket
oreille *f* ear
orteil *m* **deuxième** second toe
orteil *m* **gros** big toe
orteil *m* **petit** little toe
orteil *m* **quatrième** fourth toe
orteil *m* **troisième** third toe
oxygéner *v* to wash in peroxide; to bleach

PQ

pansement *m* plaster; dressing
parfum *m* perfume; scent; flavour
patte *f* sideburn; sideboard; side-of-face hair
paume *f* palm of hand
paupière *f* **inférieure** lower eyelid
paupière *f* **supérieure** upper eyelid
peau *f* **(grasse / sèche / sensible)** skin (greasy / dry / sensitive)
pédicurie *f* chiropody; pedicure
peigne *m* **à crêper** teaser comb
peigne *m* **à poux** fine-tooth comb (for headlice)
peigne *m* **à tige** tail comb
peigne *m* **afro; peigne africain** Afro comb
peigne *m* **à chignon** back / side comb
peigne *m* **de coiffeur** hairdresser's comb; barber's comb
peigne *m* **de coiffure** hair comb
peigne *m* **de parure** comb
peigne *m* **de poche** pocket comb
peigne *m* **fin** small-tooth comb
peigne fin *m* finishing/dressing comb
peigne *m* **soufflant; peigne sèche-cheveux** warm-air comb
peigne *m*: **coup** *m* **de peigne** comb-out
• **se donner un coup de peigne** to run a comb through one's hair
peigner *v* to comb (hair); to comb out (hair)
peigner (se) to comb one's hair

peignoir *m* cape; gown (at hairdresser's)
pellicules *fpl* dandruff
lotion *f* **contre les pellicules** anti-dandruff lotion
pendant d'oreille *f* drop earring
perçant, perçante *adj* piercing (eg of body, ears)
- **oreilles** *fpl* **percées** pierced ears

percer (se faire) *v* to pierce; to have pierced (eg ears)
permanente *f* perm; permanent wave (hair)
- **se faire faire une permanente** to have a perm / permanent wave

peroxyde *m* peroxide
perruque *f* wig; hairpiece
petrissage *m* petrissage; kneading massage
pied *m* foot
- **se faire soigner les pieds** to have a pedicure

pince *f* **à boucle de cheveux** hair curling clip
pince *f* **(à cheveux)** hairclip
pince *f* **à ongles** nail clippers
piscine *f* swimming pool
plante *f* **du pied** sole of the foot
podologie *f* chiropody; pedicure
poids *m* weight
poignet *m* wrist
poil *m* body hair
poils *mpl* **du visage** facial hair
point *m* **noir** blackhead
poitrine *f* chest; breasts; bosom
pommade *f* pomade; pomatum
pommade *f* **rosat; pommade** *f* **pour les lèvres** lip salve
pommette *f* cheekbone
porte-savon *m* soap dish
postiche *m* wig; hairpiece; toupee; piece of false hair
postiche *m* switch
postiche *m* **de cheveux** hair piece
pot *m* **de crème** pot of cream
pou m; poux *mpl* louse; lice (*pl*)
pouce *m* thumb
poudre de riz *f* face powder; rice powder
poudrier *m* powder compact
pourboire *m* tip (money)

pousser *v* to push; to grow (eg hair)
- **se laisser pousser** *v* **la barbe** to grow a beard

précoloration *f* preparation stage for colouring hair
prise *f* **(de sèche-cheveux)** hairdryer socket
produit *m* **de beauté** beauty product
produit *m* **décolorant** bleaching product
pubis *m* pubic area
pulpe *f* **de la phalangette** finger pad
pupille *f* pupil of the eye
queue *f* **de cheval** ponytail

R

racines *fpl* roots
raffermir *v* to firm up; to tone up
raide et terne *adj* lank (hair); dull (hair)
raie *f* parting (of hair)
- **porter la raie à droite/ à gauche/ au milieu** to part one's hair on the right/ left/ in the middle

rajeunissant,-e *adj* rejuvenating
ras, rase *adv*: **couper ras les cheveux** to crop the hair short or close
ras, rase *adj* close-cropped (hair, head)
rasage *m* shaving (of beard)
raser *v* to shave; to shave off
- **visage rasé** *m* clean-shaven

raser (se) *v* to shave oneself; to have a shave
- **se faire raser** to get shaved; to have a shave; to get a shave
- **se faire raser la tête** to shave one's head

rasoir *m* razor
rasoir *m* **à désépaissir** thinning razor
rasoir *m* **américain** safety razor , safety
rasoir *m* **de sûreté** safety razor
rasoir *m* **effileur** thinning razor
rasoir *m* **électrique** electric razor; electric shaver
rasoir *m* **jetable** disposable razor
rasoir *m* **mécanique** safety razor
réflexologie *f* reflexology; pressure on reflex areas of feet or hands
régénérateur *m* **des cheveux** hair restorer

régime *m* diet
régime *m* **sans graisse/ sel/ sucre** fat/ salt/ sugar-free diet
relâcher / relaxer *v* to relax
relever *v* **ses cheveux** to put one's hair up
remise en forme *v* shaping up
rendez-vous *m* appointment
repose-pieds *m* chair footrest
repousse-peaux *m* cuticle pen; cuticle remover
repousse *f* **de cheveux** hair regrowth
résille *f* hairnet
revigoré, se sentir *v* to feel refreshed
revitalisantes *adj* revitalising
ride *f* wrinkle
rinçage colorant *m* colour rinse (non-permanent)
robinet *m* **d'eau chaude / froide** tap (hot / cold)
robinet *m* **mélangeur** mixer tap
ronger (se) *v* **les ongles** bite (one's nails) (to)
rouge à lèvres *m* lipstick
• **bâton** *m* **/ tube de rouge à lèvres** lipstick; lipstick case
rougir *v* to apply blusher (eg cheeks)
rouleau (à mise en plis) *m* hair curler roller (setting roller)
rouquin, rouquine *adj* red-haired
rouquin *m*; **rouquine** *f* red-haired person; redhead
roux , cheveux red-hair; redhead

S

salon *m* **de coiffure pour hommes** barber shop
salon *m* **de coiffure pour dames** hairdressing salon
sauna *m* sauna
savon *m* soap
séchage rapide *m* hair drying (finger dry)
sèche-cheveux *m* hand dryer
séchoir *m* hairdrier; salon swivel dryer
sein *m* breast
serre-tête *m* hairband
serum *m* serum
serviette *f* **(de toilette)** towel

serviette *f* **de bain**   bath towel
serviette *f* **de maquillage**   make-up gown
serviette *f* **de toilette pour sécher**   towel for drying hair
serviette *f* **pour compresses / faciales**   towel for face compresses
shampooing *m*   shampoo
shampooing *m* **doux**   soft shampoo; gentle acting shampoo
shampooing *m* **et coupe** *f*   shampoo and cut
shampooing *m* **et mise en plis**   shampoo and set
shampooing *m* **herbal ou aux herbes**   herbal shampoo
shampooing sec *m*   dry shampoo
shampooing traitant *m*   medicated shampoo treatment
- **faire / donner un shampooing à quelqu'un**   to shampoo someone's hair
- **se faire un shampooing**   to shampoo one's hair
- **se faire faire un shampooing**   to have one's hair shampooed

shampouiner *v*   to shampoo
shampouineur *m*; **shampouineuse** *f*   shampooer (person)
shiatsu *m*   shiatsu; Japanese needleless acupuncture; massage method
soin *m*   care
soin *m* **(complet) du visage**   facial
soin *m* **des mains**   manicure
soins *mpl* **corporels; soins du corps**   body care
soins *mpl* **de beauté**   beauty treatment; beauty care
soins *mpl* **de cheveu**   haircare
soins *mpl* **de la peau**   body care
soins *mpl* **de visage**   facial
soins *mpl* **esthétiques**   beauty care
soins *mpl* **protection (couleur / perm)**   nutritive cream treatment for coloured /   permed hair
solarium *m*   solarium
soluté *m*   solution (chemical; pharmaceutical)
sombre *adj*   dark (in colour)
sommet de la tête *m* **(see crâne)**   top / crown of head
sourcil *m*   eyebrow
station *f* **thermale**   spa
stick *m* **: déodorant en stick**   deodorant stick
stick à raser *m*   shaving stick
stonethérapie *f*   stones on body's energy points
sueur *f*   perspiration / sweat

T

table de maquillage *f*   make-up table
tabouret *m*   foot stool
tache *f*   spot / pimple
tache *f* **de naissance**   birthmark
tache *f* **de rousseur / de son**   freckle
taille *f*   size; waist; waistline
taille *f* **de cheveux**   haircut; hair-cutting
tailler *v* **: se faire tailler les cheveux**   to have a haircut
talon *m*   heel of foot
tatouage *m*   tattoo; tattooing
teigne *f* tinea; scalp disease
teigne *f* **pelade; alopécie** *f*   alopecia
teindre (se) *v*   to dye one's hair
tempe *f*   temple (head)
couleur *f* **temporaire**   semi-permanent colour
thalassothérapie *f*   general sea water treatment
thermal,-e *adj*   thermal
thermalisme *m*   balneology; medically prescribed (21 day) cure
tondeuse *f*   trimmer (on electric razor)
tondeuse *f* **électrique**   electric clippers (hair)
tondre *v*   to clip (hair)
tondre *v* quelqu'un   to clip or crop someone's hair
tonique *m*   hair tonic; toning lotion
torsader *v*   to coil (hair)
touching *v*   roots colour touch-up
traitement *m*   treatment
transpiration *f*   perspiration; sweat; perspiring
tressage *m*   plaiting; braiding (US)
tresse *f*   plait
tresser *v*   to plait; to braid (US)
trousse *f* **de manucure; trousse à ongles**   manicure set; manicure case
trousse *f* **de maquillage**   make-up bag / purse
tube *m* **de crème**   tube of cream
tube *m* **de produit décolorant**   bleach tube

UV

ustensiles *mpl* **de coiffure** hairdresser's tools
vernis *m* **à ongles** nail varnish
vertiges *mpl* dizziness
vibrisse *f* nostril hair
visage *m* face

HADLEY PAGER INFO PUBLICATIONS

All publications listed are French-English and English-French

CONCISE DICTIONARY OF HOUSE BUILDING (Arranged by Trades)

Paperback, 2005 Third Edition, 304 pages, 210 x 144 mm
ISBN 978-1-872739-11-3   Price: £27.00

- Dictionary is divided into 14 sections covering the various stages and trades employed in house building: Architect, Earthworks and Foundations, Builder, Carpenter and Joiner, Woods and Veneers, Roofer, Ironmonger, Metals, Plumber, Glazier, Electrician, Plasterer, Painter and Decorator, Colours.
- Over 10.000 terms in each language. The book is the ideal companion when liaising with tradespeople or when visiting builders' merchants and DIY stores

GLOSSARY OF HOUSE PURCHASE AND RENOVATION TERMS

Paperback, 2000, Fourth Edition, 56 pages, 210 x 148 mm
ISBN 978-1-872739-08-3   Price: £7.50

- Provides over 2000 French words and phrases used by estate agents, notaires, mortgage lenders, builders, decorators, etc.

GLOSSARY OF FRENCH LEGAL TERMS

Paperback, 1999, 114 pages, 210 x 148 mm
ISBN 978-1-872739-07-6   Price: £12.00

- Provides over 4000 French legal words and phrases associated with legislation falling within the Civil Code and the Penal Code, (eg house purchase and wills), but company and commercial legislation is not covered.

GLOSSARY OF GARDENING AND HORTICULTURAL TERMS

Paperback, 2004, Third Edition, 72 pages, 210 x 148 mm
ISBN 978-1-872739-14-4   Price: £8.50

- The glossary includes nearly 2000 gardening and horticultural terms
- The glossary matches up the familiar French and English names of pot and garden flowering plants and shrubs which are not readily available elsewhere.

CONVERSATIONAL FRENCH MADE EASY
By Monique Jackman

Paperback 2005, 256 pages, 210 x 145 mm
ISBN 978-1-872739-15-1   Price £9.95

- Ideal for those with a basic knowledge of French who wish to improve and enhance their conversational skills. Particularly useful for those who have recently moved to France or have a second home there
- The book covers some 120 French verbs with more than one meaning in French. The parallel French and English translations make working alone possible, or in pairs or groups of.family members and friends

HADLEY PAGER INFO PUBLICATIONS

HADLEY'S CONVERSATIONAL FRENCH PHRASE BOOK

Paperback, 1997, 256 pages, 148 x 105 mm
ISBN 978-1-872739-05-2   Price: £6.00

- Over 2000 French/English phrases and 2000 English/French phrases
- Eleven conversational topic vocabularies. Aide-memoire key word dictionary

HADLEY'S FRENCH MOTORING PHRASE BOOK & DICTIONARY

Paperback, 2001, 176 pages, 148 x 105 mm
ISBN 978-1-872739-09-0   Price: £6.00

- Asking the Way, Road Signs, Car Hire, Parking, Breakdowns, Accidents, Types of
- Vehicle, Cycling and Motor Sports. Dictionary. Over 3000 words and phrases included

GLOSSARY OF MEDICAL, HEALTH AND PHARMACY TERMS

Paperback, 2003, First Edition, 203 pages, 210 x 148 mm
ISBN 978-1-872739-12-0   Price: £12.50

- Provides over 3000 medical, health and pharmacy terms, including common illnesses and diseases, anatomical, first-aid and hospital terms. Brief aide-memoire definitions
- Pharmacy terms include medicines, toiletries, cosmetics, health and pharmaceuticals

HADLEY'S FRENCH MEDICAL PHRASE BOOK

By Susan Kirkham and Alan Lindsey
Paperback. 2004, 156 pages, 148 x 105 mm
ISBN 978-1-872739-13-7   Price £6.00

- Invaluable to travellers in France or in the UK seeking medical advice or medical treatment Topics included are At the Doctor's, At the Hospital, Baby's, Children's, Young People's, Male and Female Health. Also At the Chemist's, At the Dentisi, At the Optician's, Accidents and •Emergencies.
- A Reference section is also included

GLOSSARY OF VETERINARY TERMS

By Susan Kirkham
Paperback. 2004, 204 pages, 210 x 148 mm
ISBN 978-1-872739-17-5   Price £14.00

- Invaluable for pet owners living in or visiting France. Over 3000 words and phrases

Hadley Pager publications are available through good booksellers or can be obtained directly from Hadley Pager Info by sending a cheque to cover the price
(postage is free within the UK, add 10% if outside the UK) to
Hadley Pager Info, PO Box 249, Leatherhead, KT23 3WX, England.

Web Site: www.hadleypager.com
Latest Publication List available on request.   Email: hpinfo@aol.com